ES
VITA

Phillip Day

 Credence Publications

The Essential Guide to Vitamin D

Copyright © 2010
Phillip Day

The right of Phillip Day to be identified as the Author of the Work has been asserted by him in accordance with the Copyright, Designs and Patents Act 1988.

Print history
First print 2010

Caution: Please note that the information contained in this booklet is for educational purposes only and should not be construed as medical advice. A properly qualified physician should always be consulted in the matter of serious illness.

ISBN 1-904015-25-5

Manufactured in Great Britain
Credence Publications
PO Box 3
TONBRIDGE
Kent TN12 9ZY UK
www.credence.org

1st ed

TABLE OF CONTENTS

"Current research has implicated vitamin D deficiency as a major factor in the pathology of at least 17 varieties of cancer as well as heart disease, stroke, hypertension, autoimmune diseases, diabetes, depression, chronic pain, osteoarthritis, osteoporosis, muscle weakness, muscle wasting, birth defects, periodontal disease, and more." – **Dr John Cannell, The Vitamin D Council**

"Because vitamin D is so cheap and so clearly reduces all-cause mortality, I can say this with great certainty: Vitamin D represents the single most cost-effective medical intervention in the United States." - **Dr. Greg Plotnikoff, Medical Director, Penny George Institute for Health and Healing, Abbott Northwestern Hospital in Minneapolis.**

"Sunlight is more powerful than any drug; it is safe, effective, and available free of charge. If it could be patented, it would be hyped as the greatest medical breakthrough in history. It's that good." – **Mike Adams, author**

"This is like the Holy Grail of cancer medicine; vitamin D produced a drop in cancer rates greater than that for quitting smoking, or indeed any other countermeasure in existence." - **Dennis Mangan, clinical laboratory scientist**

"In all my many years of practice of medicine, I've never seen one vitamin, even vitamin C, have such profound effects on human health." – **Dr Soram Khalsa, board-certified internist and medical director for the East-West Medical Research Institute**

"Vitamin D insufficiency and deficiency is a worldwide public health problem in both developed and developing nations.... Nearly one billion people worldwide are deficient." - **EurekaAlert**

INTRODUCTION

Welcome to what I consider to be one of Credence's most pivotal briefing packs. Over the past 26 years that I have reported on health matters, scarcely a more fundamental issue has come across my desk than the new scientific research on vitamin D. By way of review, vitamin D has historically been sidelined as a nutrient whose deficiencies promulgated the old medieval problems such as soft bones, rickets and osteoporosis. In the last two years, however, stunning studies have completely changed our understanding of what this nutrient is, how it works in the body, how it works in synergy with other elements, and what the implications are both for its deficiency and optimisation.

This booklet is a useful round-up of what the experts are currently saying about vitamin D. Our study here will also open up the microcosm of the human condition; the incredible intricacies of the cell; the relationship of light to human health; how the body has been uniquely designed to process sunlight in optimal amounts to prevent disease and even fix us when we are sick. Hopefully among the useful insights you will take away from this booklet will be a humble appreciation of how intricately ordered and finely tuned our Earthly condition is, and what we can do to enhance not only our own health and wellbeing, but those of our loved ones and friends who will listen. Read on and be amazed.

Phillip

NOTHING NEW UNDER THE SUN

"The whole aim of practical politics is to keep the populace alarmed - and hence clamorous to be led to safety - by menacing it with an endless series of hobgoblins, all of them imaginary." – **HL Mencken**

Most people know the sun is beneficial, though you would be forgiven for thinking the opposite with all the scare stories abounding in the media. In fact, I use my common sense as a port of first resort, and I've done this for years and have rarely slipped up. My simple maxim today is to do the complete opposite of whatever the BBC tells me to do. Why? Because I judge any expert on his results, by which means half the so-called 'health czars' of the western world should be in Guantanamo Bay zipped up in orange suits for all the disease, death and lamentations they have sown into our modern world.

Most of us are not born sceptics but we have worked out by now that politicians lie, fiddle their expenses and do immoral things. So do scientists, doctors, generals, prime ministers, weather-men, the media and just about every public servant vying to be the first to stuff their hand into our pockets. It's not that we don't want to trust our experts, it's just become a strange old world out there; a harsher, more regulated, militant, bullying, punishing playground, wherein citizens are losing control of their lives to the state, and the old safeguards of honour, morals, decency and integrity no longer apply. Welcome to the new socialist ghetto of values relativism, a New World Order wherein it is no longer enough to place your newspaper and plastic into separate containers, *you* are the problem.

'Progress' these days is all about money and selling the public on fear and 'consensus science', which is rich given that consensus is politics not science. Science either is or it isn't – that's the great thing about science. If you're not sure what the science is telling you, don't shoot your mouth off. Shut up, go back to the laboratory and run the numbers again until everyone's getting what you're getting. This drives the relativists mad. To them there is no such thing as absolute truth because it gives them no wriggle-room. Suddenly what's true

4

for you isn't necessarily true for me. Today's general denial of absolute truth is behind the greatest public health disaster of our modern age – hence the reason for this booklet.

Our 'professional' establishment comprises the same people who don't train our doctors in nutrition because they can't make any money out of it. As a consequence, these quacks have managed to make Britain the heart disease and cancer capital of the developed world while spending more per capita on healthcare than anyone else in the solar system. That takes some doing. In fact, this scandal has hit the news again as I write this – somewhat of a miracle in itself[1] - but the public is too apathetic to care. These are the same experts, by the way, who scared the pants off everyone with 'infectious' AIDS, SARS and swine flu scams to flog us dangerous drugs and vaccines we didn't need,[2] and then quietly filed these 'epidemics' away when the public got suspicious. The very same luminaries who routinely give mind-altering drugs to our kiddies based on bogus psychiatric diagnoses with no science to back them up.[3] The same people who kill our elderly with 'patient-centred senior care' involving anti-depressants, chemotherapy, radiotherapy and enough painkillers to stun a medium-sized dinosaur. The same people who told us thirty years ago the world was about to plunge into an ice age, who since changed their minds after watching Al Gore's laughable film,[4] and now pay their mortgages saying the complete opposite, namely that CO_2 is the enemy of humanity (when water vapour is by far the most prevalent greenhouse gas,

---

[1]   www.dailymail.co.uk/news/article-1234276/Britain-sick-man-Europe-Heart-cancer -survival-rates-worst-developed-world.html

[2] **Ransom, Steven & Phillip Day** *The Truth About HIV,* Credence, 2005

[3] **Day, Phillip** *The Mind Game,* Credence, 2003

[4] In 2007, a British High Court judge ruled that there were nine serious scientific 'errors' in Gore's film, *An Inconvenient Truth,* and that it was needlessly 'alarmist'. Al Gore has an established track record of exaggerating. At the Copenhagen Climate Change Conference in December 2009, he claimed a study predicted that the North Pole had a 75% chance of being free of ice by the middle of the next decade. Yet the study's author, Dr Wieslaw Maslowski, said his research revealed 'nothing of the sort': *"I would never estimate likelihood at anything as exact as this. It's unclear how this was arrived at." Daily Mail,* 16th December 2009, p.6

but you can't tax clouds), and that farting cows will be the planet's apocalypse.[5]

And then there's the sun. The reality is, the world's been going through a warming cycle since the 1940's due to increased solar output. That the sun behaves like this cyclically is well known to science, but politicians with an agenda can torture the data and get it to confess to anything. For your information, there was a macro warming period between 800-1200AD. In the 800-900s, the Vikings were farming on Greenland, which is why they called it 'Greenland', and surpluses were being exported to Scandinavia and Dublin. A hundred years later, one of the most decisive battles in English history, the Battle of Stamford Bridge, was won by King Harold II against Harald Sigurdsson ('Hardrada') of Norway, specifically because Hardrada's invading Norse had left their armour and heavy equipment with their fleet at Riccall because of the intense heat. That was on 25th September 1066, three weeks before the English army perished at Hastings.

Peter Atkinson of Ashford complains:

"The Met Office has just announced that this decade is the warmest since records began. Recent events beg the questions: Which records? When did they begin? Who provided them? What statistical manipulation, adjustments, smoothing has been applied to them to get this result? An example of a description of warm weather comes from Samuel Pepys (before records began): 'It is strange what weather we have had all winter, no cold at all; but the ways are dusty, and the flys fly up and down and the rose bushes are full of leaves, such a time of the year as was never known in this world before here.' That was in January 1661. A hundred years later, there were ice fairs on the Thames!" [6]

Which brings us to the new culprit to be hated by environmentalists: the sun. In the 1980s, the medical industry began telling everyone the sun was dangerous and could give us cancer.

---

[5] "Farmers blocked the streets of New Zealand's capital, Wellington, yesterday in protest at plans to impose the world's first 'fart tax' on livestock flatulence", *The Guardian*, 5th September 2003

[6] *Daily Mail*, 11th December 2009, p.86

Dr John Cannell writes:

"Before the sun-scare, 90% of human vitamin D stores came from skin production, not diet. Large populations of pregnant women and autistic children ingesting small amounts orally, instead of generating large amounts through the skin, are novel to human brain development.[7]

In 1989, around the time autism began to rise, the American Medical Association's (AMA) Council on Scientific Affairs warned about the dangers of sun exposure, advising mothers to "keep infants out of the sun as much as possible." In 1999, when autism rates really exploded, the American Academy of Pediatrics went further, advising mothers always to keep infants out of direct sunlight, use sun-protective clothes and sunblock, and make sure children's activities minimize sunlight exposure. Quite inexplicably, they said there was "no evidence" such "rigorous sun protection" would affect vitamin D levels. By 2002, the Centers for Disease Control (CDC) reported such efforts were quite successful: "protection from sun exposure is reported for a high proportion of children."[8]

Considerable effort was expended burbling the myth into our ears from every news bulletin, magazine article, newspaper health section and doctor's surgery noticeboard: *The sun can kill you*. At no time did the American Medical Association warn the public that vitamin D is manufactured from the sun and that levels in the population would inevitably crash if this new advice was heeded. In fact, under advice from the American Academy of Pediatrics, the recommended daily allowance (RDA) for vitamin D was actually *halved* from 400ius to 200ius despite fierce opposition from Dr Frank Greer, Professor of Paediatrics at Wisconsin University. It's instructive to note that only when people began taking the sun-scare seriously and drastically reduced their exposure to sunlight did we start to see a dramatic rise in the whole rack of serious illnesses we'll review in this booklet, most notably cancer.

---

[7] **Holick MF** "High prevalence of vitamin D inadequacy and implications for health", *Mayo Clin Proc*. 2006 Mar;81(3):353-73
[8] www.vitamindcouncil.org/health/autism/role-of-sunlight.shtml

AN AMAZING DISCOVERY

"There is a principle which is a bar against all information, which is proof against all argument, and which cannot fail to keep man in everlasting ignorance. That principle is condemnation without investigation." – **William Paley (1743-1805)**

So what about the sun? Let's sketch in some background. Wikipedia gives us the standard schoolbook excursion:

"The Sun is the star at the center of the Solar System. The Sun has a diameter of about 1,392,000 kilometres (865,000 mi) (about 109 Earths), and by itself accounts for about 99.86% of the Solar System's mass; the remainder consists of the planets (including Earth), asteroids, meteoroids, comets, and dust in orbit. About three-fourths of the Sun's mass consists of hydrogen, most of the rest is helium. Less than 2% consists of other elements, including iron, oxygen, carbon, neon, and others."[9]

The traditional scientific belief was that the universe had always existed. This was overturned once we had a proper understanding of the first three laws of thermodynamics:

1) Conservation of Energy - matter cannot be created or destroyed

2) Entropy - all systems in the observable universe are winding down (which means they used to be wound up)

3) Zero Point - if the temperature of an empty container is lowered to absolute zero (−273.15°C), there still remains a residual amount of thermal energy that cannot be removed. This is known as 'zero-point energy'

Dr Chuck Missler writes:

"Heat always flows from hot bodies to cold bodies. If the universe were infinitely old, then the temperature throughout the universe would be uniform. It's obviously not, so the universe cannot be infinitely old. This is a simple demonstration that the universe had a beginning." [10]

---

[9] www.wikipedia.org, 'sun'
[10] www.khouse.org

In other words, the universe cannot be eternal since it would have suffered ultimate heat death long before now and be of a uniform temperature. The universe is not only not a uniform temperature, it gives every appearance of still expanding and stabilising, pointing to a far more recent origin.[11] Astronomer Edwin Hubble clarified the picture when he discovered other galaxies outside our own Milky Way. He noticed that the degree of redshift observed in the light emitting from these celestial bodies increased in proportion to their distance from the observer (Hubble's Law). The impact this discovery had on science cannot be overstated. Hubble had shown that the universe had to have had a beginning and was therefore *finite.*

A combination of models was then put forward to explain how the universe could have come about. These have collectively come to be known as the Big Bang Theory which, in a nutshell, states that first there was nothing and then it exploded, and from that we got the sun, moon and stars, all highly organised by blind random chance, and everything after that too the same way, and I mean everything – newts, amoebas, rhinos, bumblebees, swans and Lady GaGa. All this stuff came from nowhere, violating Law No.1, and then evolved from simple to incredibly complex by blind random chance, apparently, violating Law No. 2. And here we are today and everything somehow just *works*. Good luck with that theory.

Since then, there's been a war going on across the sciences – chance versus design, evolution versus creation, order versus cacophony, call it what you will. This war is important for us to understand, and not necessarily for religious reasons, for it controls the type of information we get from the myriad sources we rely on for the truth. Evolutionary theory, for instance, is the reason why doctors use drugs to combat illness instead of nutrition. This catastrophic wrong turn has condemned millions to a painful, premature death.[12] So why is sunlight up for the high-jump?

---

[11] **Day, Phillip** *Origins,* Credence, 2009
[12] Ibid.

Through a glass darkly

Astronomer Dr Guillermo Gonzalez of Iowa State University enjoyed an unimpeachable career, during which he discovered several planets and was a member of NASA's astrobiology program. One event he witnessed, however, was to cause Dr Gonzalez's career to hit the skids and spin off in an entirely new direction. The trouble was caused by the publication of *The Privileged Planet,* a book he co-authored with Jay Richards. The event in question was a total eclipse of the sun the famous astronomer witnessed in Northern India on 24th October 1995.

As the moon passed across the face of the sun in the classic cosmic ballet, Dr Gonzalez experienced the marvel felt by many of his peers in the centuries preceding – that for a total eclipse to be possible, the sun, moon and Earth have to be precisely aligned in such a way that the moon's diameter perfectly eclipses the sun. Then an odd thought assailed Gonzalez. *Science just accepts that this happens without considering the odds.* What are the chances that our moon appears the same size as the sun from the Earth? Is it mere coincidence that the sun is 400 times bigger than the moon yet 400 times further away? Whoops.

The Privileged Planet eventually cost Gonzalez his job and unleashed a torrent of loathing in the scientific community against him. Interestingly, Gonzalez has never looked back. His book and film of the same name have captured the imagination of millions, revealing the science behind the anthropic principle, namely that literally dozens of incredibly fine-tuned conditions have to exist for life, or indeed the Earth itself, to be possible. Gonzalez's heresy? Earth's existence could not have come about by mere chance.

For instance, the size of the moon and its orbit are finely calibrated to stabilise the Earth's rotational angle at a 23.5°. Gonzalez realised that if the moon were a little further in, the tides would swamp the continents. A little further out and the Earth would wander off-orbit. Coincidence? If the sun were smaller or larger, the circumstellar habitable zone of our solar system would change, and if Earth did not move with it, no life would be possible, yet here we are. Earth's distance from its parent star is finely calibrated and critical. 5% closer and the atmosphere would be boiled off in the heat and Earth's rotation halted. Half the planet would roast while the other half remained in perpetual darkness and ice. 20% further away and the oceans would freeze.

It just so happens that Earth is in the optimal position in the solar system from which to observe a total eclipse. Gonzalez made a study of the other planets and moons in our system and found that the best place to observe a total solar eclipse is from the surface of the only planet which hosts complex life capable of observing and remarking on it! Of the 70-odd planets and moons (excluding Earth), only seven have atmospheres, all opaque, to whom the universe is invisible and unknown. Only Earth has a special, low-carbon, transparent atmosphere which, apart from hosting just the right chemical mix to allow life to flourish on the surface (coincidence), permits the correct UV wavelengths to reach the planet's surface from which humans can make vitamin D (more coincidence), and enables observers on the planet to gaze through its sheen into the universe beyond (even more coincidence). This facility is also only made possible *due to the Earth's precise positioning* in the Milky Way galaxy – as it happens, in the galactic habitable zone between two spiral arms from which is afforded a dust-free view into deep space. What luck!

Then there's the Earth's magnetic field which, it so happens, is just right, generated from the rotating molten iron core of the planet. The field acts as a protective shield around the Earth to ward off solar radiation which would otherwise kill us. If the size of the Earth were smaller, the magnetic field would be weaker and the solar winds would strip off the atmosphere, transforming our planet into a barren rock. Any stronger and the magnetic field would kill all life on Earth.

Many other factors have the same criticality. The weak nuclear force, the strong nuclear force, the planet's albedo (reflectivity), Boltzmann's Constant, proton and electron mass, atomic mass, speed of light, gravity, Planck's Constant, the list goes on. All these factors have to be present and fine-tuned at precisely the same time and place for life to be possible on Earth, or anywhere else for that matter, *and this still does not get you life from non-living matter in the first place.* And then there's the surprise part, say Gonzalez and Richards:

"The same narrow circumstances that allow us to exist also provide us with the best overall setting for making scientific discoveries."[13]

Earth is the only planet found so far with liquid water in abundance, critical for the sustenance of life and accurate regulation of the surface temperature of the planet. The oxygen-nitrogen mix of the atmosphere is precisely right for carbon-based life-forms to thrive in solar light. It just so happens also that our paper-thin atmosphere provides climate with which to water plants and humans, so here we are, all perfectly done. Despite his evolutionary stance, co-discoverer of DNA, Francis Crick remarked:

"An honest man, armed with all the knowledge available to us now, could only state that in some sense, the origin of life appears at the moment to be almost a miracle, so many are the conditions which would have had to have been satisfied to get it going."[14]

The flash spectrum

A total eclipse of the sun leaves a tiny disc around the edge of the phenomenon in the 51 seconds of totality, during which electromagnetic emissions from the sun's chromosphere can be observed without blinding the viewer. This unique opportunity is *only* afforded by the precise dimensions of the sun and moon. A percentage or two difference in measurement either way and stellar astrophysics would never have left the stables. As it is, studying the sun's chromosphere during a total eclipse gave us the electromagnetic spectrum, and from that we can deduce how other stars and planets work and how life itself came to be possible.

A study of the electromagnetic band given off by our sun's chromosphere – the flash spectrum – reveals another miracle. Namely that within the vast band of solar radiation emitted by our

---

[13] **Richards, Jay W and Guillermo Gonzalez** *The Privileged Planet,* Regnery, 2004
[14] **Crick, F** *Life Itself: Its Origin and Nature,* Simon and Schuster, New York, 1981, p.88

sun, which ranges from gamma through x-ray to ultraviolet to infrared, microwave and radio, there exists an impossibly narrow zone of visible light in the middle, by which all things live and can be seen. This visible spectrum comprises *only 1 trillion of a trillionth* of the entire range of the universe's electromagnetic emissions! And imagine that this just so happens to be the light spectrum our sun emits in abundance, containing UVA and UVB, which can penetrate our wafer-thin atmosphere in precise amounts to be used by plants, animals and humans for photosynthesis and life. *"It's a surprise,"* says Gonzalez. *"It's something you wouldn't expect just chance to produce."*[15]

In my book *Origins,* I cover these and many other stunning discoveries which are forcing a complete re-think of how we got here and the nature of the powers which sustain us. Remember, inherent in the theory of evolution is the complete denial of any organising intelligence/input, which flatly contradicts Watson and Crick's discovery of the four-nucleotide alphabet on DNA, which is *digital information.* Where did that come from? DNA is a three-out-of-four, error-correcting digital code containing start and stop bits to parse the assembly instructions for every protein of every living organism on Earth. Put another way, the same software is being used to make and sustain every living creature in our world. More than that, the entire system on Earth is operating synergistically and simultaneously with innumerable sub-systems at multiple levels of sophistication far beyond our comprehension in stunning assemblage and ordered arrays. And at the heart of how it all works is the sun.

---

[15] *The Privileged Planet* documentary, www.illustramedia.com

THE VITAMIN D MIRACLE

"Humans make thousands of units of vitamin D within minutes of whole body exposure to sunlight. From what we know of nature, it is unlikely such a system evolved by chance."
- **John J Cannell MD, Executive Director, Vitamin D Council**

Everyone knows the sun is essential to human health except Professor Karol Sikora. Take a plant and shut it up in a cupboard and you know what happens. Sunlight is essential for life and although widely acknowledged, science is less enthusiastic about discussing *the type of light* we get in such abundance for the reasons covered in the previous chapter. The other reason science hates the sun is because the public can get the golden globe's benefits for nothing, so there's no profit. What other reason can you come up with for medicine's continued *refusal* to trumpet bold new initiatives for prescribing sunlight after the amazing studies published over the past five years? John Maher, DC, DCCN, FAAIM, comments:

"Natural sunlight's benefits are not limited to vitamin D production. As light enters the eyes, photoreceptors convert the light into nerve impulses that travel along the optic nerve to the brain. These impulses trigger the hypothalamus gland to send neurotransmitters to regulate the automatic functions of the body, such as blood pressure, body temperature, respiration, digestion, sexual function, moods, immune and hormonal modulation, and circadian rhythm."[16]

Recent studies show that sunlight is so vital to human health that vitamin D alone up-regulates about 10% of the human genome. Vitamin D is made from the sun in humans by the action of solar radiation acting on the cholesterol of our skin to produce the nutrient. Vitamin D's usable derivative is technically not a vitamin but a secosteroidal, oil-soluble hormone. Dr Joseph Mercola provides the technical summary:

"The sun is the source of UVA and UVB. UVB is used to make vitamin D. Four UVB protons combine with one molecule of cholesterol

---

[16] www.vitamindcouncil.org

(7-DHC), opening a ring to make vitamin D3. The liver converts vitamin D3 to 25(OH)D3 [calcidiol]. Virtually all epithelial tissues convert it to 1,25(OH)2D3 [calcitriol]."[17]

The vitamin D system is elegant and sophisticated. Two hydroxylation processes must occur before arriving at the final form, 1,25-dihydroxycholecalciferol, which is more commonly known as calcitriol. Both UVA and UVB radiation are absorbed by us but have very different characteristics. Only UVB can make vitamin D3. UVA destroys it. Far from being a curse, the proper application of both types of UV to human skin is necessary and actually provides a check and balance system to prevent over-production of vitamin D.

The Vitamin D Council reports that:

"The high rate of natural production of vitamin D3 cholecalciferol (pronounced koh ·luh ·kal ·sif ·uh ·rawl) in the skin is the single most important fact every person should know about vitamin D—a fact that has profound implications for the natural human condition.

Technically not a 'vitamin', vitamin D is in a class by itself. Its metabolic product, calcitriol, is actually a secosteroid hormone that targets over 2000 genes (about 10% of the human genome) in the human body. Current research has implicated vitamin D deficiency as a major factor in the pathology of at least 17 varieties of cancer as well as heart disease, stroke, hypertension, autoimmune diseases, diabetes, depression, chronic pain, osteoarthritis, osteoporosis, muscle weakness, muscle wasting, birth defects, periodontal disease, and more.

Vitamin D's influence on key biological functions vital to one's health and well-being mandates that vitamin D no longer be ignored by the healthcare industry, nor by individuals striving to achieve and maintain a greater state of health."[18]

---

[17] www.mercola.com, vitamin D resource center
[18] www.vitamindcouncil.org

Simple to complex?

The human body is incredibly complex, consisting of upwards of 40-50 trillion cells. In Darwin's day, the limits of science prevented any meaningful studies into the smallest structures, so the idea that a homogenous glob comprising the first cell might have been mankind's earliest ancestor – a simple life-form from which extraordinary complexity derived – was accepted with nary a blush, no proof given. Biologist Thomas Huxley, known as 'Darwin's Bulldog', wrote:

> "Looking back through the prodigious vista of the past, I find no record of the commencement of life, and therefore I am devoid of any means of forming a definite conclusion… but… if it were given to me to look beyond the abyss of geologically recorded time to the still more remote period when the Earth was passing through physical and chemical conditions, which it can no more see again than a man recall his infancy, I should expect to be a witness of the evolution of living protoplasm from not-living matter."[19]

Even today, the blithe assumption is made that living matter evolved from non-living matter. This is no small matter, neither is it science. After World War 2, the cell began to be unlocked with the advancement in technology unavailable in Charles Darwin's day. What confronted scientists down the new electron microscope, however, was not Charlie's homogenous glob of undifferentiated protoplasm, but a miniaturised city of untold complexity containing molecular machines performing numerous tasks. Professor of Biochemistry, Michael Behe, writes:

> "At the very basis of life where molecules and cells run the show, we've discovered machines, literally molecular machines… There are little molecular trucks that carry supplies from one end of the cell to the other. There are machines which capture the energy from sunlight and turn it into usable energy…. When we look at these machines, we ask ourselves,

---

[19] **Huxley, Thomas** "Biogenesis and Abiogenesis", *Collected Essays of T H Huxley,* (1894) Macmillan and Co, London, 1970

where do they come from? And the standard answer – Darwinian evolution – is very inadequate in my view."[20]

Even the 'simplest' cells are now known to be unbelievably complex. Biochemists have tabulated their components – mitochondria, nucleus, rough endoplasmic reticulum, Golgi apparatus, cytoskeleton, smooth endoplasmic reticulum, proteins, fats, enzymes, minerals, and so on – but not the *biophysical* aspects the cell, which include the ability to process sunlight and organize the information required to assemble and replicate the cell, not to mention the bizarre property of one cell being able to communicate with others over distance.[21] Dr Missler writes:

"The 'simple cell' turns out to be a miniaturized city of unparalleled complexity and adaptive design, including automated assembly plants and processing units featuring robot machines (protein molecules with as many as 3,000 atoms each in three-dimensional configurations), manufacturing hundreds of thousands of specific types of products. The system design exploits artificial languages and decoding systems, memory banks for information storage, elegant control systems regulating the automated assembly of components, error correction techniques and proof-reading devices for quality control."[22]

And running this incredible show? On a molecular level, sunlight, water, nutrients and air, the very essentials markedly absent from your doctor's medical training roster. In fact, your doctor was trained is evolutionary, Descartian/Newtonian biochemistry – actually pharmacology – and was given little to no understanding of any part of the human metabolic picture. Perhaps he attended one lecture on nutrition if he wasn't playing golf that afternoon. The result? 21st century Earth is enduring an unprecedented public health catastrophe because those we trusted refuse to go where the evidence led because there was no gold at the end of the rainbow. The public too colludes in its own destruction

[20] *Unlocking the Mystery of Life* DVD, www.illustramedia.com
[21] **Stone, Robert B** *The Secret Life of Your Cells*, Whitford Press, 1989
[22] **Missler, Chuck** *In the Beginning, There was Information*, audio presentation supplementary notes, Koinonia House, www.khouse.org

by swallowing everything Nurse shoves down its throat without demur. W Deutscher summed up this state of affairs in a course handout at the University of Manchester Institute of Science and Technology, remarking:

"We concentrate on consistency without much concern of what it is we are being consistent about, or whether we are consistently right or wrong. As a consequence, we have been learning a great deal about how to follow an incorrect cause with the maximum of precision."

THE GREAT PUBLIC HEALTH DISASTER

"My parents warned me never to open the cellar door or I would see things I shouldn't see. So one day when they were out I did open the cellar door and I did see things I shouldn't see – grass, flowers, the sun…." – **Emo Phillips**

We've made some great advances in medicine, who would argue? Infant survivability at birth? Brilliant. A & E trauma medicine? Brilliant. God forbid you cut your leg off with a lawnmower, they're very good at sticking it back on again. You might die of MRSA in the process but at least you'll die with both legs on, so don't complain. Pain management? Brilliant. Prosthesis? Brilliant. Transplants? Not bad at all. Disease? *Pathetic.* Mental health? *Don't get me started.*

My point? It serves you to know what doctors are good at doing and where they are hopeless. Doctors are hopeless at disease if they refuse to accept that patients are the sum total of everything they've ever done to themselves, and that they can be fixed the same way. It's obvious when you think about it, and it doesn't get more basic than food, water, sunlight, exercise, air and lack of stress. Not getting that list sorted is what's killing everyone. Many doctors bridle and call it alternative health but, really, how alternative is food and sunlight?

And on the subject of sunlight, how much we get is a downright prerequisite for health. Birds make vitamin D from the action of sunlight on their feathers, then they preen themselves and ingest the vitamin D. Mammals such as cats get their vitamin D from the UV action on their fur, from which the nutrient is made and then licked off by the animal. That doesn't mean you've got to go round licking cats in the sun, just appreciate that important changes in human existence have occurred in the past century which have upset the fundamentals of how our health is maintained. And everyone's paying a terrible price.

For instance, unlike our forebears, who spent a great deal of time outdoors invading foreign countries, today it's common to spend 40 hours a week in an office playing *Call of Duty*. And then there's time spent in the car or on a train or plane. For several years I worked in an office in Vauxhall, London, which necessitated my leaving home fifty miles away in Kent to catch the train to London. Once the clocks went back from October onwards, I'd get up in the dark and walk to the local station in the dark. When I got to London, dawn was but a smudge in the sky. I'd walk in the gloom the mile to my office and once inside, no subsequent sunlight penetrated that hideous edifice.

I worked under artificial light. Come 1pm, it was an orange juice and salad for lunch down in the canteen, then back up the grim high-rise until after dark. At 5pm, I'd walk back to station in the dark, catch the train home in the dark, stumble up my garden path in the dark, and that Sisyphean day repeated itself from October to March, during which time the only sun I ever saw was in the travel agent's window I passed outside Waterloo East by the hotdog stand.

Location, location, location

Another big problem is where we live. Sunlight's wavelength changes the further north we dwell, which means that north of the 52^0 parallel, you're not making vitamin D from equinox to equinox. Grab a map and you'll see that the 52^0 parallel runs across the southern reaches of Canada, ten miles above Cork, Ireland, through Milton Keynes, UK, and crosses the European coastline south of The Hague. Again, nature's made allowances, granting people who traditionally live in these northern climes a fairer skin, which creates vitamin D efficiently from the paucity of UV available. Thus Irish and Scottish folk are characterised by fair/pale skin, whereas Africans have deeply pigmented skin, enabling them to spend more time outdoors without damage. Evolutionists posit that these traits came about by natural selection acting on random variations over hundreds of thousands – even millions of years. The problem is, we've only got 6.7 billion people on the planet. If you do a simple compound maths exercise in your next tea-break, you'll discover mankind's been in the sex business for around 4,400 – 5,000 years, *not millions*. All right, I'll give you 7,000 or even 10,000 years, taking into account wars, plagues, etc. Not nearly enough time for natural selection acting on random variations to wreak its charm. What do we actually observe? The ethnic/skin profiles of populations were ideally suited to their respective, indigenous climates before we began flying and sailing everywhere.

Now introduce multiculturalism, stir up the populations and see what happens. Take large numbers of African Americans and dump them in Detroit, Chicago, Cleveland and Minneapolis. Take thousands of Afghans, Iranians, Iraqis and Saudis and get them to live north of the Watford Gap in the UK. Naturally, permit all Muslim women to wrap themselves up according to their custom so they receive no sunlight which, let's face it, they wouldn't be getting in Leicester anyway even if they were Katie Price. What is the outcome? Thousands of sick, vitamin-D-deficient African Americans in Chicago and Detroit, and multitudes of sick, vitamin-D-deficient Afghans, Iranians, Iraqis and Saudis going to the National Health Service for help, whereupon the latter gives them drugs, ex-chemical warfare agents (chemo) and radiation for their cancers, and Prozac for their depression. No-one mentions sunlight because the whole subject of skin colour is racist, and don't ye know that the sun's killing the planet?

Cancer

I've studied cancer for 26 years, done countless talks and tours on the subject all over the world, appeared on TV and radio, written books. There's no doubt that we've seen substantial progress in *orthomolecular medicine* (therapeutic nutrition) against all forms of the cancer while the orthodox lot are still about their cut, slash and burn. The shameful truth is, for all the billions spent, the five-year or better survival rates for almost all forms of cancer have remained unchanged for the past forty years in our regular oncology units, hence the grim headlines in today's newspapers.[23] This is not only a scandal, it's a crime. All the good news about nutrition, mycology, dehydration, acidosis and toxicity relating to cancer has been a

---

[23] *Daily Mail*, "Britain, the sick man of Europe: Heart and cancer survival rates among worst in developed world", 9th December 2009

matter of peer-reviewed, public record for the past sixty years, yet completely ignored because the answers don't pay. I get challenged on this all the time by doctors who write me withering emails. That's right, the same doctors who are shovelling sugar into their cancer patients after they've knocked them flat with chemotherapy, ask whether I'm serious about implying that doctors would willingly withhold a cure for cancer if they knew something worked! Like I'm oft fond of saying, you can be sincere, and you can be sincerely wrong.

These professionals have the same Internet access as I do so they are without excuse. To be fair, many of them know that if they did start treating their cancer patients metabolically, their career would be over faster than a ferret up a trouser leg. The good news is, there are many ex-patients walking around *properly* free of cancer today due in no small part to the patient learning for themselves about the condition, taking control and changing their diet and lifestyle accordingly. They are sometimes confronted by their physicians for doing this, threatened with dismissal, cajoled, ignored, shouted at, and if a child with cancer is in the middle, proceedings can be undertaken to have the minor forcibly removed from their parents by court order for compulsory 'treatment' (poisoning/irradiation). If the child subsequently dies, the doctor has immunity from prosecution.

In spite of this, I've seen the tremendous benefits of alkalising, organic raw diets, plenty of exercise, detoxing, vitamins B17, C-complex, A&E, and a slew of antifungals on all forms of cancer. Only in the last 36 months, however, has empirical evidence emerged over what I consider to be the missing link with cancer on the cellular level – and that is sunshine and the marvellous action of vitamin D.

In Dr Joseph Mercola's book, *Dark Deception – Discover the Truth About the Benefits of Sunlight,* the famous internet doctor covers vitamin D's role in cancer prevention and treatment in detail. In his online talk on vitamin D, he shows charts which reveal how geographically sensitive cancer incidence is – for example, when plotted for latitude.[24] Britain's cancer chief, Professor Karol Sikora, couldn't care less. His 'impassioned' pleas on behalf of British cancer patients mention nothing about vitamin D, not one word on nutrition, and merely lament why cancer 'victims' are not being given the right drugs because of their postcode.[25]

What about the dozens of studies now in the literature which show that optimal sunlight reduces incidences of breast cancer, colon, prostate, lung (early-stage) Non-Hodgkin's lymphoma and melanoma?[26] That optimising vitamin D levels in their cancer patients and cleaning up their diet/lifestyle should be the first thing to which an oncologist sets his hand? That vitamin D is thought to work by improving cell differentiation, apoptosis (death of rogue cells), boosting immunity and reducing inflammation? That optimising vitamin D levels not only prevents someone getting cancer in the first place but boosts their chances of overcoming the disease in treatment? A list of these studies can be viewed in detail at www.vitamindcouncil.org/researchCancer.shtml. Don't take my word for it. Your life, or the life of someone you love, could be at stake because of the continued lock-down of this information.

---

[24] www.mercola.com, search under 'vitamin d'

[25] *Daily Mail*, 20th November 2009

[26] **Boscoe, FP & Schymura, MJ** *BMC Cancer*, 10;6;264, November 2006; *Crit Rev Oncol Hematol*. 2009 May 13

WHAT'S VITAMIN D GOOD FOR?

"It has been clearly established that the only way for your body to synthesize vitamin D is in your skin once it's exposed to ultraviolet rays from the sun. Hence, the current guidelines to avoid sun exposure, and the fervent pushing of sunscreen, are perhaps some of the most misguided and dangerous health recommendations out there." **- Leif Grunseth, neuromuscular consultant**

One question I always get asked when I tour Down Under is, 'If sunlight's so good for us in Australia, why is there a skin cancer clinic on every corner?' Good question. As previously mentioned, the idea that the sun causes cancer – specifically skin cancer – was promulgated aggressively in the 1980s by the medical profession. The message? Stay out of the sun and slather carcinogenic sunblock/creams all over your body instead. Studies show that skin cancer incidence began to increase significantly only after this nonsense was implemented and, might I add, on the heels of 100 years of monitoring skin cancer incidence with little appreciable increase during that period. So, two questions:

1) Were there always skin cancer clinics on every corner in Australia? No.

2) Why did incidences of skin cancer skyrocket from the point when people actually began *decreasing* their sun exposure by staying out of the sun? Two reasons: one, vitamin D levels in the population crashed and two, most sunscreens not only contain carcinogenic chemicals, most lotions actually filter out UVB while allowing in UVA. The net result is that no vitamin D is made and UVA is the UV component that actually damages the skin, causing skin cancer. Sunscreens providing 'Sun Protection Factor 8' reduce vitamin D synthesis by 97.5% while SPF 15 nails it by 99.9%. Not good.

Dr Mercola reports that skin cancers can also be caused by an over-consumption of omega-6 fats (polyunsaturated vegetable fats). Changing the ratio of omega-3s to -6s in the diet is also a problem, as are transfats which increase free radical damage. Add to that a commensurate decrease in consumption of raw fruits, veggies and other antioxidant foods in favour of processed foods and the picture becomes bleaker.[27]

Naturally, no-one's making the claim that barbecuing your flesh won't cause skin cancer, but it's only half the story. Dr William Grant believes that 200,000-300,000 Americans die each year from cancers generated from vitamin D deficiency in an effort to avoid 1,500 deaths from sun-induced skin cancer, many of which wouldn't occur in the first place if the patient was vitamin-D-optimised and didn't fry themselves. To put this into perspective, "...*for every death from skin cancer due to excess UV, more than 200 die from all cancers due to insufficient UV,*" says Dr Mercola.[28]

Clearly sunburn is dangerous and no-one's pretending otherwise. What most don't realise is that while sunburn increases melanoma risk (creating a healing process which does not terminate), prudent exposure to sunlight *reduces* melanoma risk by 15%, not only because of the vitamin D produced, but because UV is deadly to the cellular fermentation processes and fungal proliferation upon which melanoma depends to spread.

Summary of vitamin D research

Those seeking more information on the following conditions and their link with vitamin D deficiency should start their homework at www.vitamindcouncil.org and work outward from there. Other excellent websites are given at the end of this booklet to round out your research. There's nothing but good news to be had from optimising your vitamin D levels. It's cheap to do and you have nothing to lose.

---

[27] www.mercola.com, search under 'vitamin d'
[28] Ibid.

Vitamin D deficiency conditions

CANCER:[29] Bladder, brain, breast,[30] colon and rectal,[31] endometrial, eye, liver, lung, lymph, melanoma, pancreas, skin and prostate[32]

AUTO-IMMUNE:[33] Lupus, hypo/hyperthyroidism (Graves), diabetes types-1/2[34], multiple sclerosis[35], rheumatoid arthritis, Sjogren's syndrome, ankylosing spondylitis, inflammatory bowel disease (Crohn's), coeliac disease, parathyroid function, psoriasis, sarcoidosis

CARDIOVASCULAR: Chronic obstructive pulmonary disease (COPD), hypertension, stroke

NERVOUS/NEUROMUSCULAR: Addison's, cerebral palsy, epilepsy, migraine, muscular weakness, neuralgia, chronic pain, Parkinson's[36]

---

[29] **Hansen CM, Binderup L, Hamberg KJ** "Vitamin D and cancer: effects of 1,25(OH)2D3 and its analogs on growth control and tumorigenesis", *Front Biosci.* 2001 Jul 1;6:D820-48.

[30] **Grant WB** "An ecologic study of dietary and solar ultraviolet-B links to breast carcinoma mortality rates", *Cancer* 2002 Jan 1;94(1):272-81

[31] **Platz EA, Hankinson SE, Hollis BW** "Plasma 1,25-dihydroxy- and 25-hydroxyvitamin D and adenomatous polyps of the distal colorectum", *Cancer Epidemiol Biomarkers Prev.* 2000 Oct;9(10):1059-65

[32] **Polek TC, Weigel NL** "Vitamin D and prostate cancer", *J Androl.* 2002 Jan-Feb;23(1):9-17; **Tuohimaa P, Lyakhovich A, Aksenov N** "Vitamin D and prostate cancer", *J Steroid Biochem Mol Biol.* 2001 Jan-Mar;76(1-5):125-34

[33] **Panda DK, Miao D, Tremblay ML** "Targeted ablation of the 25-hydroxyvitamin D 1alpha-hydroxylase enzyme: evidence for skeletal, reproductive, and immune dysfunction", *Proc Natl Acad Sci USA,* 2001 Jun 19;98(13):7498-503; **Deluca HF, Cantorna MT** "Vitamin D: its role and uses in immunology", *FASEB J.* 2001 Dec;15(14):2579-85

[34] **Hypponen E, Laara E, Reunanen A** "Intake of vitamin D and risk of type 1 diabetes: a birth-cohort study", *Lancet* 2001 Nov 3;358(9292):1500-3; **Billaudel B, Barakat L, Faure-Dussert A** "Vitamin D3 deficiency and alterations of glucose metabolism in rat endocrine pancreas", *Diabetes Metab* 1998;24:344-50

[35] **Hayes CE** "Vitamin D: a natural inhibitor of multiple sclerosis", *Proc Nutr Soc.* 2000 Nov;59(4):531-5; **McMichael AJ, Hall AJ** "Multiple sclerosis and ultraviolet radiation: time to shed more light", *Neuroepidemiology,* 2001 Aug;20(3):165-7

[36] **Evatt ML, Delong MR, Khazai N, Rosen A, Triche S, Tangpricha V** "Prevalence of vitamin D insufficiency in patients with Parkinson's disease and Alzheimer's disease", *Arch Neurol.* 2008 Oct;65(10):1348-52

GENETIC: Cystic fibrosis, sickle cell, Turner's syndrome

ENDOCRINE: PMS[37], Syndrome X

MENTAL: Depression, schizophrenia, seasonal affective disorder,[38] Alzheimer's,[39] autism

JOINT/BONE/SKELETAL: Osteoarthritis,[40] osteoporosis, osteomalacia, osteopenia, otosclerosis, rickets, hip fractures

INFECTIOUS: Influenza,[41] colds, pneumonia, upper respiratory tract infections, urinary tract infections, etc. Vitamin D is a potent antibiotic which increases antimicrobial peptides. 100 years ago, tuberculosis was effectively managed used sunlight and decent nutrition

MISC: Asthma,[42] general gastrointestinal,[43] miscarriage, PMS, renal function, eczema, insomnia, hearing loss, periodontal disease, age-related macular degeneration, myopia, pre-eclampsia, infertility, breast-fed babies with vitamin-D-deficient breast milk, obesity[44]

---

[37] **Thys-Jacobs S** "Micronutrients and the premenstrual syndrome: the case for calcium", *J.Am.Coll.Nutr.* 2000;19:220-7

[38] **Gloth FM 3rd, Alam W, Hollis B** "Vitamin D vs broad spectrum phototherapy in the treatment of seasonal affective disorder", *J Nutr Health Aging.* 1999;3(1):5-7

[39] **Masoumi A, Goldenson B, Ghirmai S et al** "1alpha,25-dihydroxyvitamin D3 interacts with curcuminoids to stimulate amyloid-beta clearance by macrophages of Alzheimer's disease patients", *J Alzheimers Dis.* 2009 May 11; **Oudshoorn C, Mattace-Raso FU, van der Velde N, Colin EM, van der Cammen TJ** "Higher serum vitamin D3 levels are associated with better cognitive test performance in patients with Alzheimer's disease", *Dement Geriatr Cogn Disord.* 2008;25(6):539-43. Epub 2008 May 26

[40] **McAlindon TE, Felson DT, et al.** "Relation of dietary intake and serum levels of vitamin D to progression of osteoarthritis of the knee among participants in the Framingham Study", *Ann Intern Med* 1996; 125: 353-359; **Lane NE, Nevitt MC, Gore LR, Cummings SR** "Serum levels of vitamin D and hip osteoarthritis in elderly women: a longitudinal study", *Arthritis Rheum* 1997; 40(suppl): S238

[41] **Cannell JJ, Vieth R, Umhau JC, Holick MF et al** "Epidemic influenza and vitamin D (Review)", *Epidemiol Infect.* 2006 Dec;134(6):1129-40. Epub 2006 Sep 7

[42] **Clifford RL, Knox AJ** "Vitamin D - a new treatment for airway remodelling in asthma?" *Br J Pharmacol.* 2009 Nov;158(6):1426-8

[43] **Ghezzi A, Zaffaroni M** "Neurological manifestations of gastrointestinal disorders, with particular reference to the differential diagnosis of multiple sclerosis", *Neurol Sci* 2001 Nov;22 Suppl 2:S117-22

[44] **Wortsman J, Matsuoka LY, Chen TC, Lu Z, Holick MF** "Decreased bioavailability of vitamin D in obesity", *Am J Clin Nutr.* 2000 Sep;72(3):690-3)

VITAMIN D DOSAGE AND TESTING

Have you ever read an article which says, "Vitamin C is useless"? Did you ever wonder why one week vitamin C seems to be saving the world and the next it's killing everyone? Once again there's a war underway and the public mind is the pawn and the prize. Every time I think I've become immune to all the rubbish put out by government and science departments during my career, I realise I haven't. Generals lie to protect their rear-ends. Bankers lie to make money. Politicians lie to get re-elected, bribed or buy a duck house. Scientists lie to get renewed tenure and grants.[45] Doctors lie to make money and avoid prosecution. Caught in the middle of it all, Joe Public blinks like the rabbit in the headlights, paying for it all, perishing every day from Deutscher's entrenched error when, for a ha'porth of care and interest, those Joe believed actually gave a darn refused to tell him how not to die of a disease not even Joe's farm animals were dying from.

The big deal about vitamins

Almost all trials which show little or no efficacy with vitamins are low-dose studies. Did you ever wonder how these substances came to attract the vitamin label in the first place? The term 'vitamin' was originally coined in the early 19th century from a contraction of the words 'vital' and 'mineral'. The definition has progressed since, and can be regarded as an organic compound whose deficiency will cause an illness, every time, without question. Take 50 people and suck all the vitamin C out of them and 50 people will get scurvy. The problem is measurable, empirical. A sub-category of vitamin classification might be, 'an essential compound for health which cannot be synthesized by an organism and thus must be procured from diet.' I'm not so fond of that one since most

---

[45] *Times Online,* "One in seven scientists say colleagues fake data", 4th June 2009, www.timesonline.co.uk/tol/news/science/article6425036.ece

mammals can make vitamin C in their bodies and it's still a vitamin. Anyway, the Free Dictionary classifies a vitamin as:

"…any of a group of substances that are essential in small quantities for the normal functioning of metabolism in the body. They cannot usually be synthesized in the body but they occur naturally in certain foods: insufficient supply of any particular vitamin results in a deficiency disease."[46]

The good news is, vitamins prevent disease and they can cure disease. While this may be hotly contended by the Food and Drug Administration and its pharmaceutically bribed clones around the world, the medical literature is replete with the studies.[47] It's common sense when you think about it. The deficiency of the item which causes scurvy (ascorbate) will cure scurvy if the compound is returned to the diet. What cures prevents, and what prevents cures. This is true for a range of metabolic illnesses from scurvy to beriberi to pernicious anaemia to pellagra (sometimes schizophrenia), and it's the same for vitamin-D-deficiency problems.

RDAs

Science produces recommended daily allowances (RDA) for vitamins which are supposed to be the minimum amounts required to prevent an overt deficiency disease. But, as Professor Ian Brighthope of Melbourne points out, if you give every Australian the RDA of vitamin C (60 mg), you still see scurvy.[48] This is because vitamins don't work in isolation but are actioned synergistically in the body along with their metabolic co-factors. A complicated interaction of factors can influence how much of a nutrient is available for use by the body. Stress, for instance, depletes vitamin C because stress produces adrenalin, and for every molecule of adrenalin produced, you sacrifice a molecule of vitamin C as the catalyst. The result? Vitamin requirements vary per individual so

---

46 www.thefreedictionary.com/vitamin
47 www.orthomolecular.org
48 www.foodmatters.tv

RDAs are meaningless. Moreover, RDAs have nothing to do with a vitamin's...

Therapeutic range

This is the dosage at which stuff gets done. Let's take a common example. Give everyone 120 mg of vitamin C (twice the RDA) and nothing happens. Actually something *does* happen. The individual *probably* doesn't get scurvy, but not so you'd notice. There's therefore a difference between prevention – what you can't see happening – and therapeutic dosage, when you do see things happening, i.e. the patient gets better. This is the point missed, or probably ignored by scientists who, let's be honest, aren't going to pay their mortgages flogging vitamin C to a grateful public.

The therapeutic range of C does not really start for an average adult under 3,000 mg. Then you need to factor in when the doses are taken, how far apart they are taken and in what amounts. Sounds complicated. Vitamin C has a half-life in the body of roughly four hours,[49] so progressively loading up the blood serum with vitamin C throughout the day is far more effective than taking one load in a single shot. And there's evidence in vit C's case that only a certain amount can be used at a time by the body, so shovelling in half a trailer-load before breakfast, in vitamin C's case, is not going to be of benefit, whereas dividing the dose will be.

All vitamins have a half-life in the body, and how they work and the best way to administer them differs enormously. As we'll see in a minute, vitamin D's half-life is a bit more impressive and its application is about as straightforward and inexpensive as it gets. You just need sun. Then again, if you live in England where we've not seen the sun since 1976, you might have to pay a bit more with Thomas Cook to go get some sun.

---

[49] Namely, if you take 2 g of vitamin C at breakfast, you'll only have 1 g in the system by lunch, 500 mg by tea-time, and 250 mg by supper time.

Vitamin D RDA and sun-dosing

The recommended daily allowance for vitamin D is set at 200-400 international units a day (iu). This is thought to be the level above which overt cases of the classic vitamin D deficiency disease rickets will not be observed. Alas, it's not that simple. You actually need around 4,000iu/day just to maintain the vitamin D levels you've already got. Do you think government scientists know this already? Of course they do. To understand vitamin D's playing field a little better, consider the following.

Let's say you went out to the local park in June between 11am and 2pm, stripped completely naked and laid out on the grass. In the half an hour it took for the local plod to arrest you, scientists say you can generate around 20,000iu of vitamin D. Of course, the mitigating factors are skin pigmentation, where you are on the planet, cloud cover, pollution, speed of police, etc. Then you get bailed out at the station, return home with your clothes on, strip off again for a shower...and wash all that vitamin D straight down the plughole!

That's right. It takes around 48 hours for vitamin D to penetrate the skin. Being oil-soluble, vitamin D is broken down by soap and washed away in your power shower. To avoid this happening after adequate sun exposure (enough for you fair-skinned types to turn pinkish), wash off the skin with water and tend to the underarms and groin area separately. Smelly old farmers live longer – pungent but true. Dark-skinned folk need much more sun than light-skinned folk.

Watch to see when your shadow is shorter than you are. Dr John Cannell says this is a useful thumbnail to determine when you can make vitamin D. Unfortunately in the UK, your shadow is longer than you are for a good six months of the year. Trying to get sun exposure behind glass won't work either since the vitamin-D-making UVB wavelength is disrupted. UVA gets through, however, and that's not good news.

The purpose of this booklet is to get you to take *reasonable* sun exposure not only more seriously, but to view it as one of the cardinal prerequisites for a longer life. Numerous studies indicate

31

that 'all-cause mortality' is significantly higher if you are vitamin-D-deficient.[50]

Vitamin D testing

If you have cancer or other serious condition, the first thing to do is find out what your blood serum levels of D are. You can do this even if you are healthy and just want to know. The test you should request is known as a 25(OH)D3 or 25-hydroxy D3 test for calcidiol, and is done using a blood sample. Ask for the results to be calibrated in nanograms per millilitre (ng/ml), the standard scale. If you end up with other calibrations, convert as follows:

10 ng/ml = 10µg/L (no change)
10 ng/ml = 24.96 nmol/L

The ng/ml scale runs as follows:

<30 ng/ml – deficient
60 ng/ml – normal
70-90 ng/ml – therapeutic
>100-110 ng/ml –toxic threshold

Dr Bruce Hollis remarks that no circulating D3 can be found until levels are 40-50 ng/ml. By this measure, at least 85% of the US population are vitamin-D-deficient. Consider that America is below the 52nd parallel, so the UK and northern Europe will be worse.

If your test comes back deficient, vitamin D levels should be raised using sunlight, and then a re-test a few weeks later to see if progress is being made. There are specially designed, electronic-ballast 'safe' tanning beds, too, which emit predominant UVB wavelength. Dr Mercola recommends these but they are expensive and not to everyone's tastes.[51] Your last option is vitamin D3 (cholecalciferol) supplementation, which is cheap and convenient

---

[50] www.vitamindcouncil.org/science/research/vitamin-d-and-mortality.shtml
[51] www.mercola.com

but by no means the best solution. If you are pushing the limits with supplementation, the experts advise that you to get tested often and watch for calcium levels rising – an indication of the toxic threshold.

For most people, D3 oral supplementation will be the only option, especially during winter months. Dr Mercola states that normal healthy individuals can supplement 3000iu/day per 100lbs bodyweight and for those undergoing treatment for cancer or other serious illnesses, 5000iu/day per 100lbs bodyweight. If you are pushing the limits with oral supplementation, it is vital to monitor levels not only to avoid the aforementioned overdosing, but also to ensure the therapeutic margin is gained. Some people require huge initial doses of D3 to get them into the game. You simply won't know where you stand without testing and monitoring your levels. Remember also that you weren't designed to take vitamin D orally, so you won't get all of the benefits associated with normal sun exposure, says Dr Mercola, which is by far the most safe and efficient method of vitamin D production:

"There is no way to know if the recommendations given below are correct. The ONLY way to know is to test your blood. You might need 4-5 times the amount recommended below. Ideally your blood level of 25(OH)D should be 60ng/ml." [52]

AGE	ORAL DOSAGE
Below 5	35iu per lb per day
5-10	2,500iu/day
18-30	5,000iu/day
Pregnant women	5,000iu/day

---

[52] Ibid.

FREQUENTLY ASKED QUESTIONS (FAQ)

Q: What is the half life of vitamin D in the body?

A: 4-6 weeks from the sun. 4-6 months from oral supplementation.

Q: Can I get vitamin D from my food?

A: Yes, some food does contain vitamin D but not nearly enough. You need sunlight. John Cannell MD writes:

"We get a little in our diet, almost all of it from milk or fish, but none of us get enough from our diet. We also get some in multivitamins, but multivitamins only contain 400 units, which is about 10% of the body's daily need. It appears to us that the best thing to do is be conservative and maintain natural vitamin D blood levels year-round by receiving sunlight in the summer and supplementation in the winter. In this case, 'natural' means blood calcidiol levels similar to humans living in a natural relationship with the sun, such as farmers in Puerto Rico or lifeguards in the United States. Both groups have calcidiol levels above 50 ng/ml.

So the amount an individual would need to prevent cancer really depends on how much sunlight exposure they receive in terms of duration, the time of year and time of day, and the amount of skin exposed. Any vitamin D already being received through diet and supplementation should be considered as well."[53]

Do not be fooled by so-called fortified vitamin D foods. These use a vegetable form of the nutrient, D2, *which is not human vitamin D*. Foods such as fortified soy milk, yoghurts, etc., impair your D conversion to critical hormones and block vitamin D receptors. Avoid, avoid, avoid.

Q: Are there safe sunscreens I can use?

A: Yes, Neways International does one my family and I use on holiday. See www.neways.com. Nevertheless, understand there has been much ozone layer, climate change, and sunshine

---

[53] www.vitamindcouncil.org/cancerMain.shtml

scaremongering. Appropriate exposure to the sun *free of cream/block* is what your body was designed for. *Do not barbecue your flesh.*

Q: If I mention vitamin D deficiency and the 25(OH)D3 test to my doctor, will he know what I am talking about?
A: If he doesn't, slap him, then educate him.

Q: If I am pregnant, can I supplement?
A: Yes. It is vital for mums to be tanked up for their little ones to avoid birth defects and premature births, and also afterwards to ensure the breast milk is suitably fortified. Dr Mercola recommends 5000ius/day during pregnancy. During breastfeeding, 4000-5000ius/day is safe without any evidence of toxicity or vitamin-D-related adverse effects to mother or infant.[54] Sunshine is far better than supplements if you can get it. Witness the *Times* article below:

Vitamin D 'may cut premature birth risk and protect newborn babies'

"Powerful new evidence about the way that vitamin D can reduce the risk of premature births and boost the health of newborn babies has emerged from an international research conference in Bruges. Delegates were told that mothers who were given ten times the usual dose of vitamin D during pregnancy had their risk of premature birth reduced by half and had fewer small babies.

The findings emerge after evidence, revealed in *The Times*, that vitamin D — the "sunshine vitamin" — could have a dramatic effect in combating Scotland's appalling health record. Statistics showing that Scots — particularly in the west — are exposed to less sunshine than those living farther south <u>correlate exactly with higher incidences of heart disease, some cancers and multiple sclerosis</u> [emphasis mine]. *The Times* has campaigned to have vitamin D recommended and prescribed as part of a national health programme."[55]

---

54 www.vitamindcouncil.org/research.shtml
55 www.timesonline.co.uk, 10th October 2009

Q: How important is vitamin D to my kids and should I be supplementing them?

A: Try to get them outside to do it the natural way. Failing that, sensible supplementation is advised by the proper experts. US Health Ranger, Mike Adams writes:

Sunlight deficiency is now at epidemic levels

"Kids are sunlight-deficient and that's due to a few reasons: First, too many kids today spend most of their hours in front of computers, televisions or gaming consoles. The live almost like vampires, staying awake all night, sleeping during the day, living off the flesh of other creatures (beef jerky and hamburgers...). Many of their parents, too, are part of the problem. Today's moms seem terrified that their kids might actually experience 'the outdoors' for more than a few moments. They wait with air-conditioned cars at the school bus-stops, then hustle their kids into pre-cooled cars to drive the quarter mile back to their artificially air-conditioned homes. Sunlight almost never touches these kids (they might turn to dust)."[56]

Q: What are the symptoms of vitamin D toxicity?

A: Nausea, vomiting, loss of appetite, headache, dry mouth, abdominal or bone pain, and dizziness. Elevated calcium levels are watched for by doctors, and when we speak of vitamin D toxicity, it's usually the excess calcium that's the problem. Merck reports:

"The main symptoms result from hypercalcemia. Anorexia, nausea, and vomiting can develop, often followed by polyuria, polydipsia, weakness, nervousness, pruritus, and eventually renal failure. Proteinuria, urinary casts, azotemia, and metastatic calcifications (particularly in the kidneys) can develop."[57]

Q: I'm not sick as such but do want to take my health more seriously. What can I do?

A: The regimen in the next section will give you a summary of key areas to address. In addition, have a look at our other titles which deal with a whole range of health issues in more detail.

---

[56] www.naturalnews.com/026770_Vitamin_D_health_health_care.html
[57] www.merck.com/mmpe/sec01/ch004/ch004k.html

THE *FOOD FOR THOUGHT* LIFESTYLE REGIMEN
The broad-strokes of a healthy lifestyle

➢ Little or no meat in the diet. Any meat consumed should be hormone- and pesticide-free. White meat is better than red. Avoid pork completely

➢ Avoid sugar, dairy, coffee and alcohol

➢ Ensure 80% of your diet comprises properly constituted, organic, whole, living foods, 60% of your diet should be eaten raw. Remember, heat kills enzymes and vitamin C, corrupts fats and destroys 50% of the protein. In other words, cooking destroys the information in your food

➢ Learn the art of juicing veggies which makes consuming raw foods easy and effortless

➢ If you want hot, briefly steam your veggies, do not murder them. Excellent recipes are provided in our companion guide, *Food For Thought*

➢ The ideal balance is: 80% alkali/20% acidic ash foods Most diets today comprise 90% acid/10% alkali

➢ Some broiled fish, deep and cold caught, eaten sparingly is OK

➢ Avoid the foods below

➢ Hydrate the body with 2 litres (4 pints) of clean, fresh water a day

➢ Keep high-glycaemic fruit intake down. Eat more fruits that have low sugar-conversion, such as pears and apples. Don't juice more of the fruit than you would eat of it

➢ Try to eat six *small* meals a day, ensuring a) that you don't go hungry, and b) that the body has a constant supply of nutrients. This evens out blood sugar fluctuations

➢ Set up a basic supplement program which should include ionised colloidal trace minerals, antioxidants,

vitamin C and B complexes along with essential fats and vitamin D3, where appropriate
- ➢ Exercise to assist in detoxing the body in an oxygen-rich environment. A regular walk in the early morning air is healthy and invigorating. Get the heart-rate elevated for 20-30 minutes a day. Studies show that this transforms your health
- ➢ Rest. Rest. Rest. Rest. Rest
- ➢ Reduce environmental toxicity (avoid jobs using dangerous chemicals, radiation, etc.)
- ➢ Use safe personal care products[58]
- ➢ Use safe household products[59]
- ➢ Reduce stress. If you are leading a stressful lifestyle, you need to change that lifestyle. Don't ignore this!

Foods to avoid
- ➢ Pork products (bacon, sausage, hot-dogs, luncheon meat, ham, etc.) These can contain parasites, are high in nitrites and are known homotoxins which can cause high blood urea and dikitopiprazines, leading to brain tumours and leukaemia[60]
- ➢ Scavenger meats, including ALL shellfish. Carrion-eaters - pork and shellfish in particular - concentrate toxins of other animals in their tissues, which we then consume to our detriment. The same goes for the elimination organs of commercially raised animals, such as liver and kidney, which can be high in drug and pesticide residues
- ➢ Aspartame/saccharin, artificial sweeteners. These cause known mental impairment problems and cancer risks
- ➢ Refined sugar/flour/rice. SUCROSE FEEDS CANCER Restricted amounts of wholegrain bread are OK. Use

---

[58] www.neways.com
[59] Ibid.
[60] **Day, Phillip** *Food for Thought*, Credence, 2004; **Reckeweg, HH** "Adverse influence of pork consumption on human health", *Biologic Therapy*, vol.1, no.2, 1983

only wholegrain rice. No sugars should be consumed other than those contained naturally in whole foods

> Hydrogenated & partially hydrogenated fats (margarine)
> Junk (processed) food, including fizzy sodas and other soft drinks containing sugar, artificial sweeteners or phosphoric acid, which are drunk out of aluminium cans
> Fat-free foods. Essential fats are *essential!*
> Olestra, canola, soy, etc. Avoid fake or synthetic fats and foods fortified with vitamin D2. Soy, in its unfermented state (meat and milk substitute products), disrupts the hormone (endocrine) system, blocks the absorption of calcium and magnesium, and acts like estrogen in the body
> Polluted water (chlorinated or fluoridated – see *Health Wars*, 'Water Under the Bridge')
> Caffeine products
> Alcohol products
> Excess refined salt. It's better to spice food with ground kelp to maintain a healthy iodine intake or use Himalayan salt. Half a teaspoon a day of the latter has great health benefits.[61] Remember, all your body fluids are water and salt!

For a full analysis of 'food as it should be', see *Food For Thought*, the food recipe companion to *Health Wars* and *Cancer: Why We're Still Dying to Know the Truth*

---

[61] **Batmanghelidj, F & Phillip Day** *The Essential Guide to Water and Salt,* Credence, 2008

CONCLUSION

Well, there you have it. This is not a subject you can do full justice to in forty pages, but do check out the websites in the next section and do your research on this fascinating subject. I am constantly asked what, in my view, are the leading purges of 21st century humanity. Science spends millions doing studies on this every year but after 26 years of my own research, here are the problems:

1) cooked food
2) dehydration
3) lack of sunshine
4) lack of exercise
5) too much stress
6) too much toxicity

How much control do we have over the above? 100%! That's what the Credence mission is all about. I invite you to take the time to look at our other books, CDs, DVDs and briefing packs. They are loaded with useable, lifesaving information, and like this booklet, have been designed to provide scientifically grounded answers to some of the greatest health problems we face. Also sign up for our free Internet EClub bulletins and weekly health tips (see next section).

Today can be the start of the new you with a future full of knowledge and confidence. We are so lucky. Major answers have been found to some of the greatest problems dogging humanity, and I am confident that when the public gets to hear of them, they'll run with the information and pass the word onto others. Please help by being part of that process.

Good health!

Phillip

CONTACTS! CONTACTS! CONTACTS!

If you wish to purchase more copies of this booklet or obtain any of Credence's other book, audio or video titles, please use the contact details below. Credence has local sales offices in a number of countries. Please see our website at **www.credence.org** for further details:

> **UK Orders:** (01622) 832386
> **UK Fax:** (01622) 833314
> **www.credence.org**
> **e-mail:** sales@credence.org

Obtaining health products
If you need more information or help with any of the materials discussed in this book, please use the above contact details.

Useful websites on vitamin D
www.mercola.com
www.vitamindcouncil.org
www.naturalnews.com
www.orthomolecular.org
www.doctoryourself.com

Credence Publications
PO Box 3
TONBRIDGE
Kent TN12 9ZY, UK

THE CAMPAIGN FOR TRUTH
IN MEDICINE

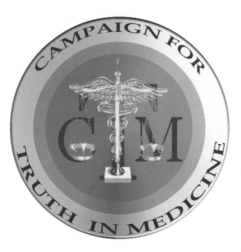

WHAT IS CTM?

The Campaign for Truth in Medicine is a worldwide organisation dedicated to educating the public on health issues and pressing for change in areas of science and medicine where entrenched scientific error, ignorance and vested interests are costing lives. Our ranks comprise doctors, scientists, researchers, biochemists, politicians, industry executives and members of the public, all of whom have come to recognise that in key areas of disease, drug treatments and healthcare philosophy, the medical, chemical and political establishments are pursuing the wrong course with the maximum of precision, even when their own scientific research has warned of the dangers of these courses.

CTM STANDS FOR CHOICE IN HEALTHCARE

Millions today use nutritional supplements and alternative health strategies for themselves and their families, yet increasingly the public's freedom to choose is being eroded by government legislation and attempts by the pharmaceutical conglomerates to 'buy out' the alternative health market. CTM stands for the people's right to choose the healthcare system they feel is right for them, free of big business interference, pointless government regulation, and coercion by the medical establishment, which often attempts to compel its own dubious remedies upon an unwilling public.

SIGN UP FOR REGULAR BULLETINS AND HEALTH TIPS!

Every month, CTM sends out EClub, its global online magazine, to keep subscribers informed of the latest news, developments, scandals and great news in healthcare and other relevant issues. Within EClub, doctors, researchers, journalists, scientists and leading healthcare advocates share their tips, views and strategies with hundreds of thousands around the world. EClub represents the news you are not being told; information that can literally change and save lives. Don't miss out on this vital resource, forwarded FREE to you every month! To join, visit credence.org.

HOW TO ORDER CREDENCE PRODUCTS

Credence has offices and distributors in many countries around the world. If you would like more information, or wish to purchase any of the Credence titles described, please use the details in the **Contacts!** section of this book. Alternatively, why not visit Credence's comprehensive web-site at **www.credence.org**, which contains secure on-line global stores, a fully searchable database and many other great features.

Please note: Items not available in your regional shop may be obtained through our default 'Rest of World' store.

ABOUT THE AUTHOR

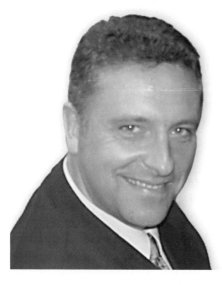

Phillip Day was born in England in 1960. He was educated at the British education establishments Selwyn and Charterhouse, and throughout his twenties had a successful entrepreneurial career founding businesses in sales and marketing. With a firm grounding in business and the ways of the media, Phillip's research career began after he became interested in wars going on in the realms of health and politics over issues that were being deliberately withheld or misreported to the public.

Phillip Day heads up the publishing and research organisation Credence, now located in many countries around the world, which collates the work provided by researchers in many fields. He is also founder of the worldwide Campaign for Truth in Medicine (CTM), whose free monthly Internet newsletter may be obtained by registering at www.credence.org. CTM's intention is to work with the establishments and organisations concerned to resolve health issues that are harmful to the public, and to provide the necessary information for citizens to make their own informed choices in these vital matters. Phillip's speaking schedule is exhaustive and takes him to audiences all over the world.

He is married to Samantha, has a daughter Anna, and lives in Kent, England.